Zepbound-Friendly Christmas Cookies

Your Favorites Made Easy

Dr. Max Noah

Table of Contents

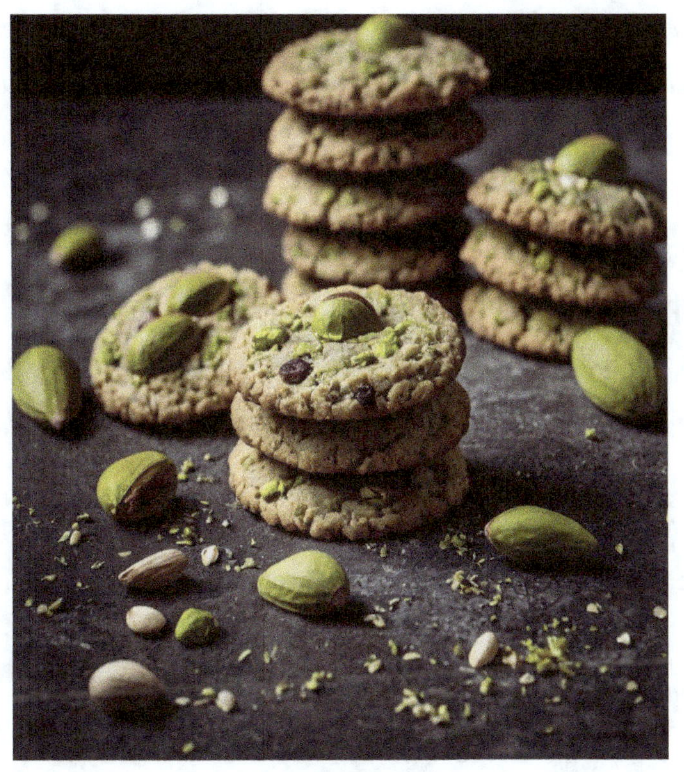

Happy Baking!

Introduction

Hey bakers! I hope you're all feeling festive and excited to whip up some cookies. I know this time of year can be hard when you're focused on your health - but never fear, because this cookie book is here!

Inside these pages you'll find all your classic holiday favorites, totally reimagined to satisfy your sweet tooth without the guilt or blood sugar spikes. Gone are the days of sacrificing flavor or texture just to keep things better-for-you.
From Gingerbread to Peanut Butter Blossoms, you'll find recipes galore to please every palate, using natural ingredients and perfect portion sizes. Just think - you can finally indulge your cookie cravings while still sticking to your Zepbound goals!

I want you all to feel included this season without compromising your wellness. So grab an apron, whip up a batch and dive on in! These cookies are guaranteed to delight whether you're prepping for parties or just need a cozy treat by the fire.

And most importantly, remember that balance is key. Enjoy the flavors and time with loved ones - your health is the greatest gift you can give yourself.

As you dive into these recipes, I hope you'll see this book as more than a collection of goodies to enjoy - it's meant to help reclaim the true meaning and comfort of this festive time.

By baking these Zepbound-friendly treats, not only will you nourish your body but also make memories with loved ones, spread holiday cheer through gifts, and develop a much healthier view of indulgence. Think beyond just the flavors - focus on the people and togetherness they represent.

So go ahead, tie on those festive aprons! We're about to embark on a cookie-filled journey that leaves you feeling merry, satisfied and proud of your wellness progress. I promise, the best gifts are the ones you feel good enjoying without compromise.

Have fun exploring both nostalgic and new finds. And remember, balance is key - savor the season, appreciate your people, feel free! Wishing you all the happiest and healthiest of holidays.

Happy baking, and may your holidays be merry and bright - one Zepbound-friendly cookie at a time!

Now, who's ready to bake?

Chapter 1: Gingerbread Squad

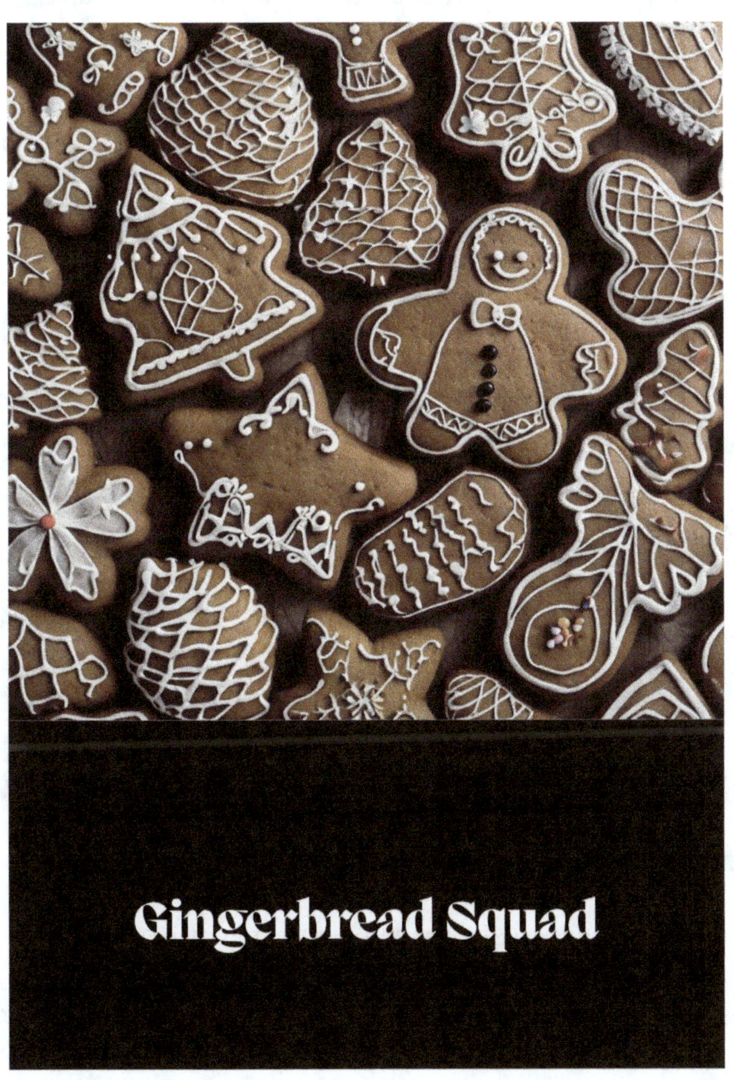

A Single-Serve Adventure!

Because sometimes you just need a couple of adorable gingerbread friends to keep you company without turning your kitchen into Santa's entire workshop!

What You'll Need (for 2 perfectly portioned cookies)

- 1/2 cup blanched almond flour (yes, blanched matters - we're fancy here!)
- 1 tablespoon monk fruit sweetener (keeping it Zepbound-friendly, wink wink)
- 1/4 teaspoon ground ginger (the spicier, the merrier!)
- 1/8 teaspoon ground cinnamon (just a cozy little pinch)
- Tiny pinch of ground cloves (we're talking TINY - these little guys pack a punch)
- Teensy pinch of salt (because even healthy cookies need personality)
- 1 tablespoon unsalted butter, melted and cooled (or coconut oil for dairy-free folks)
- 1 small egg yolk (sorry egg white, maybe next time!)
- 1/4 teaspoon vanilla extract (the real stuff - treat yourself!)

- Optional but awesome: 1 scoop (about 15g) unflavored whey protein powder

Let's Make Magic!

1. First things first - crank that oven to 325°F (165°C). We're not savages who throw cookies into cold ovens!

2. In a bowl that's just the right size (meaning whatever's clean), whisk together your almond flour, monk fruit sweetener, all those warming spices, and salt. If you're going protein-style, toss that in too. Feel free to do a little whisking dance - no one's watching!

3. In another bowl (or the same one if you're feeling rebellious and don't mind living on the edge), mix your melted butter, egg yolk, and vanilla until they're as well combined as a holiday choir.

4. Marry these two mixtures together until you've got a dough that looks like it could win a gingerbread beauty pageant. It might be a bit sticky - that's totally normal!

5. Pop this lovely dough in the fridge for about 15 minutes. Perfect time to check your socials or do those dishes you've been avoiding!

6. Line a small baking sheet with parchment paper (because who enjoys scrubbing pans? Nobody, that's who).

7. Split your chilled dough into two equal portions. Roll each into a ball, then flatten to about 1/4 inch thick. You can use a cookie cutter if you're feeling fancy, or just go rustic-style with circles. Both taste equally delicious!

8. Bake these little darlings for 10-12 minutes, or until they're just starting to get golden around the edges. Your kitchen should smell like Christmas threw a party!

9. Let them cool on the baking sheet for 5 minutes (I know it's hard to wait, but we believe in you), then transfer to a rack to cool completely.

The Numbers Game (per cookie, because math is fun!)

- Calories: 45 (or 52 with protein powder)

- Protein: 2g (5g with protein powder)

- Net Carbs: 1g

- Fat: 4g

- Fiber: 1g

- Sugar: 0g (monk fruit sweetener for the win!)

Pro Tips from Your Kitchen Bestie:

- These cookies actually get better the next day, but who are we kidding - they probably won't last that long!

- Store in an airtight container if by some miracle you don't eat them immediately

- Feel free to add a tiny sugar-free icing face if you're feeling artistic. Even grumpy gingerbread men make great company!

Remember: These aren't your grandma's sugar-bomb cookies, but they're about to become your new best friends on your Zepbound journey. Besides, who doesn't want to be able to say they have a "gingerbread squad"?

Now go forth and bake your heart out, you magnificent cookie creator!

Chapter 2: Keto Chocolate Snowballs

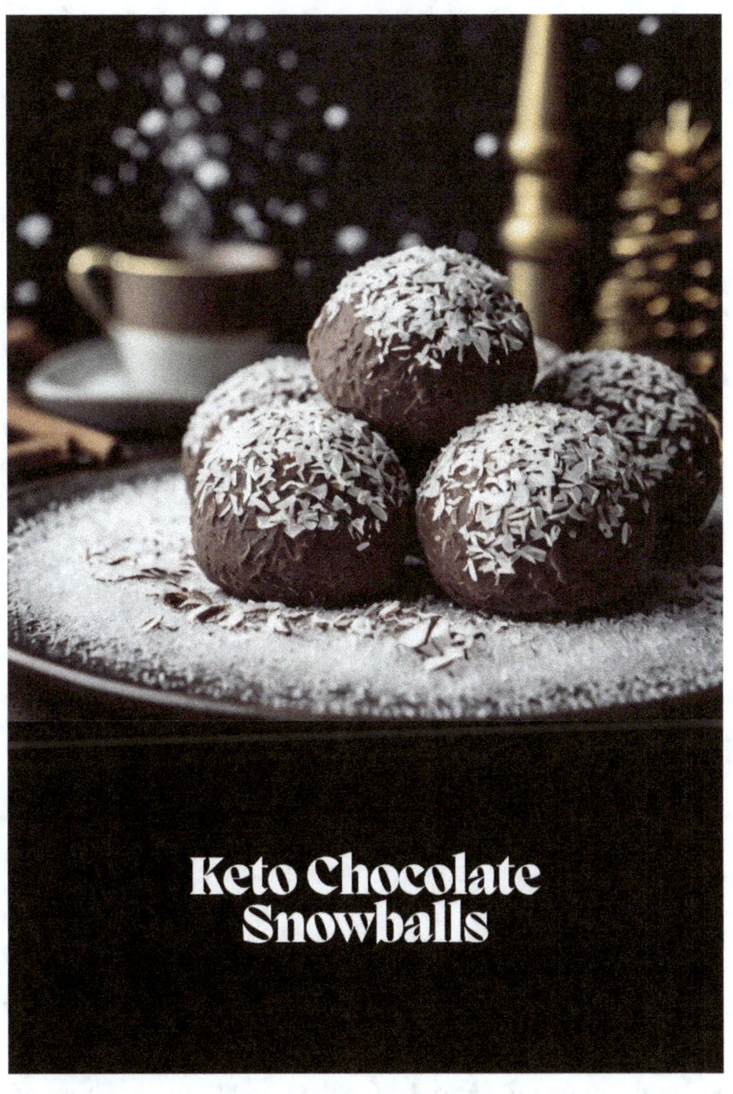

You know those moments when you're craving something chocolatey but don't want to derail your progress? Well, grab your mixing bowl because these babies are about to become your new best friend! They're like regular chocolate snowballs went to fitness camp and came back all healthy and sophisticated.

Makes: 2 servings (2 cookies per serving)
Prep Time: 15 minutes
Chill Time: 30 minutes

Ingredients:
• 3 tablespoons coconut flour (trust me, it's better than it sounds!)
• 2 tablespoons unsweetened cocoa powder (the good stuff!)
• 2 tablespoons powdered allulose (our secret weapon)
• 2 tablespoons melted butter (because we're not complete saints)
• 1 tablespoon heavy cream
• ¼ teaspoon vanilla extract (splash it in there!)
• 1 tablespoon sugar-free chocolate chips, finely chopped

• 2 tablespoons finely chopped pecans

• Extra powdered allulose for rolling (make it snow!)

For That Gorgeous Snowy Coating:

• 2 tablespoons powdered allulose

Instructions (Let's Make Some Magic!):

1. First things first - grab a medium bowl and mix your coconut flour, cocoa powder, and powdered allulose. Give it a good whisk like you're conducting a tiny orchestra!

2. Now, pour in that melted butter, heavy cream, and vanilla extract. Mix until it looks like chocolate playdough. If it's too dry, add a tiny splash of cream. Too wet? A pinch more coconut flour will do the trick!

3. Fold in those chopped chocolate chips and pecans. This is where the magic happens, folks!

4. Time to get your hands dirty! Roll the mixture into 4 equal-sized balls. Think ping-pong ball size, not bowling ball!

5. Here comes the fun part - roll these little guys in the extra powdered allulose until they look like they've been caught in a snowstorm.

6. Pop them in the fridge for about 30 minutes. Perfect time to catch up on that show everyone's been talking about!

Storage Tip (Because Willpower Is Hard):
Store the extras in an airtight container in the fridge for up to 5 days. But let's be honest, they probably won't last that long!

Nutritional Information (per serving - 2 cookies):
• Calories: 65 per cookie (130 total per serving)
• Fat: 6g
• Net Carbs: 2g
• Fiber: 2g

• Protein: 2g

• Sugar Alcohols: 3g

Pro Tips From Someone Who's Been There:

1. Don't skip the chilling time - these little guys need their beauty rest!

2. If your hands get too sticky while rolling, wet them slightly with cold water.

3. Keep these stored in the fridge - they're better cold anyway!

Remember: Just because you're on Zepbound doesn't mean you can't have your cookie and eat it too! These little snowballs are proof that healthy eating doesn't have to taste like cardboard.

Chapter 3: Protein-Packed Holiday Snickerdoodles

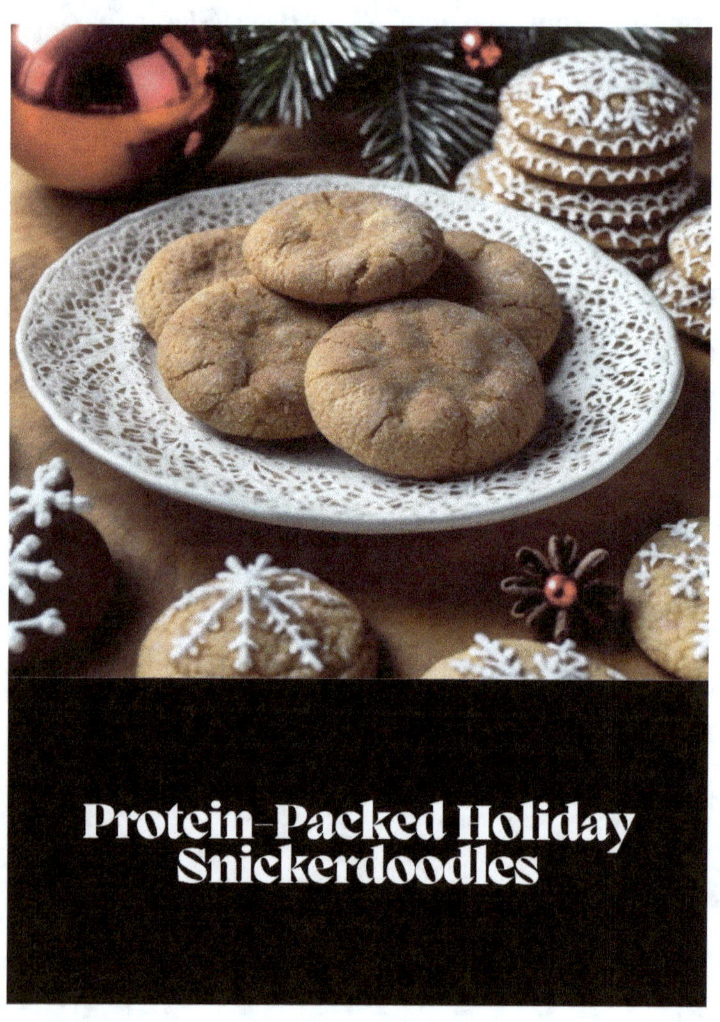

Makes 2 servings (4 cookies total)

Listen, if you're like me and think regular snickerdoodles are basically a vehicle for cinnamon-sugar happiness, you're in for a treat! These protein-packed cookies will give you all the cozy vibes without the sugar crash. Plus, they're Zepbound-friendly!

Ingredients

<u>For the Cookies:</u>

- 1 scoop (30g) vanilla whey protein powder

- 3 tablespoons (21g) blanched almond flour

- 1 tablespoon (12g) monk fruit sweetener

- ¼ teaspoon baking powder

- Tiny pinch of salt (trust me on this!)

- 1 large egg white

- 1 tablespoon unsweetened almond milk

- ¼ teaspoon vanilla extract

- Optional but recommended: ⅛ teaspoon butter extract (it's our little secret!)

<u>For the Cinnamon Coating:</u>

- 1 teaspoon monk fruit sweetener

- ½ teaspoon ground cinnamon

- Pinch of nutmeg (optional, but adds that extra holiday magic)

Instructions:

1. Preheat your oven to 350°F (175°C). Line a small baking sheet with parchment paper. (No parchment? A little cooking spray will do in a pinch!)

2. In a small bowl, mix your cinnamon coating ingredients. Set aside and try not to sniff it too much – it smells like Christmas!

3. In a medium bowl, whisk together your protein powder, almond flour, sweetener, baking powder, and salt. Break up any lumps – we're going for smooth cookie bliss here!

4. In a separate small bowl, whisk your egg white until slightly frothy (about 30 seconds). Add almond milk and extracts.

5. Here comes the magic: Pour your wet ingredients into the dry ingredients. Mix until you get a soft dough. If it seems too dry, add a tiny splash more almond milk. Too wet? Sprinkle more almond flour. We're looking for a dough that's just right – Goldilocks would approve!

6. Divide the dough into 4 equal portions and roll into balls. Roll each ball in your cinnamon coating mixture until well covered. Place on your prepared baking sheet and gently press down to flatten slightly. (They won't spread much during baking.)

7. Bake for 8-10 minutes, or until the edges are just set but the middle is still slightly soft. Don't overbake! We want cookies, not frisbees.

8. Let cool on the baking sheet for 5 minutes (I know it's hard to wait, but your fingers will thank me), then transfer to a wire rack to cool completely.

Storage Tips:

Store in an airtight container for up to 3 days, if they last that long! You can also freeze them for up to a month – perfect for emergency cookie cravings.

Nutritional Information (per 2-cookie serving):

- Calories: 100
- Protein: 12g
- Net Carbs: 3g
- Fat: 4g
- Fiber: 1g
- Sugar: 0g

Pro Tips:

- Let's be real: protein cookies can be tricky! If your first batch isn't perfect, don't worry. Adjust the liquid slightly next time.

- These are best enjoyed slightly warm (15 seconds in the microwave works wonders!)
- Pair with your favorite sugar-free hot chocolate for maximum holiday vibes
- Perfect for leaving out for Santa if he's watching his macros this year!

Remember: Life is too short for bad cookies, but too precious for cookies that don't love us back. These little gems do both!

Chapter 4: Sugar-Free Thumbprint Cookies

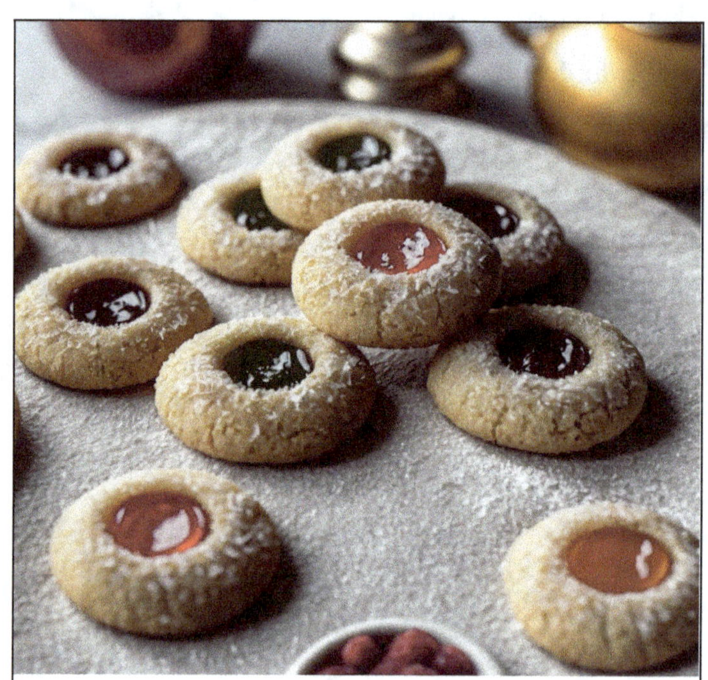

You know what's better than a cookie? A cookie with a little jammy surprise in the middle! This recipe makes just 4 adorable cookies, perfect for when you want a treat without having dozens tempting you from the cookie jar.

Ingredients:
• 1/2 cup coconut flour
• 2 tablespoons softened butter (trust me, room temp is key unless you want an arm workout!)
• 2 tablespoons monk fruit sweetener (because we're sweet enough already)
• 1 small egg white
• 1/4 teaspoon almond extract (our secret weapon for that bakery-style flavor)
• 1/8 teaspoon vanilla extract
• Pinch of salt (just a tiny hello of sodium)
• 2 teaspoons sugar-free raspberry jam (or whatever jam rocks your world)
• Optional: 1 tablespoon finely chopped almonds for rolling

Instructions:

1. First things first - crank that oven to 325°F (165°C). Line a small baking sheet with parchment paper because nobody likes cleanup duty!

2. In a small bowl, cream together your butter and sweetener until it's fluffy and living its best life (about 2 minutes).

3. Add that egg white and your extracts - mix until everything's partying together nicely.

4. Gradually stir in the coconut flour and salt. The dough might look a bit crumbly at first (don't panic - this is normal!). Let it sit for 2 minutes to let the coconut flour do its thing and absorb moisture.

5. Roll into 4 balls (about 1.5 inches each). If using nuts, roll the balls in the chopped almonds now.

6. Place on your prepared baking sheet and make a thumbprint in each cookie (hence the name - genius,

right?). Pro tip: use the back of a teaspoon if you want to keep your thumb clean!

7. Fill each depression with about 1/2 teaspoon of sugar-free jam. Don't go overboard - we're not making jam tarts here!

8. Pop these babies in the oven for 12-15 minutes or until the edges are just slightly golden brown.

9. Let them cool on the baking sheet for 5 minutes (I know it's hard to wait, but your fingers will thank you), then transfer to a cooling rack.

Nutritional Info (Per Cookie):
• Calories: 55
• Protein: 1.5g
• Net Carbs: 2g
• Fat: 4.5g
• Fiber: 3g

Storage Tips:

These little gems will keep in an airtight container for 3 days, but let's be honest - they rarely last that long!

And there you have it, my friend! A perfectly portioned batch of thumbprint cookies that won't throw your Zepbound journey off track. They're so good, you might find yourself doing a little happy dance in your kitchen. But hey, I won't judge - that just means extra calories burned!

Remember: The best thing about this recipe is that it makes just enough to satisfy your sweet tooth without having extras calling your name at midnight. Because we all know those midnight cookie cravings are REAL!

Chapter 5: Sugar-Free Peppermint Chocolate Meringues

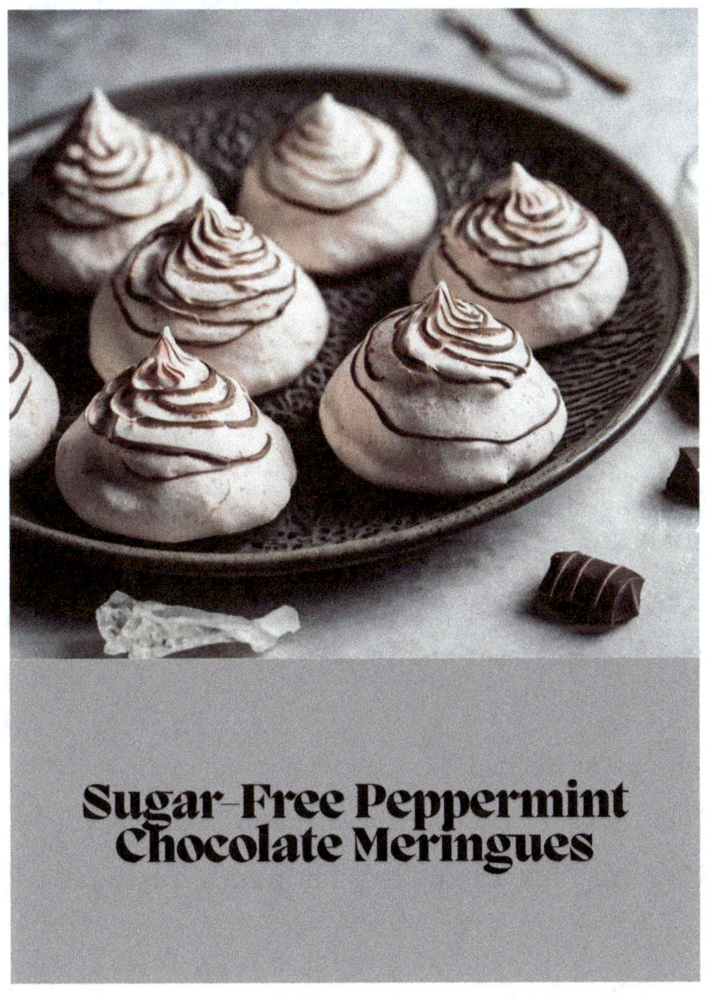

Makes 6-8 small meringues (perfect for 1-2 people)

Listen, I know what you're thinking - "Sugar-free meringues? Is that even possible?" Well, grab your mixing bowl and prepare to be amazed! These little clouds of joy are about to become your new favorite Zepbound-friendly treat.

Ingredients

- 1 large egg white (room temperature is crucial!)
- 3 tablespoons allulose or monk fruit sweetener
- 1/8 teaspoon cream of tartar (your egg white's best friend)
- 1/4 teaspoon pure peppermint extract
- 2 tablespoons sugar-free mini chocolate chips
- Pinch of salt (just a tiny one!)

Equipment Needed

- Hand mixer or stand mixer (your arm will thank you)
- Clean, dry mixing bowl (any hint of grease is the enemy!)
- Parchment paper

- Piping bag or zip-top bag (for fancy points)

Instructions

1. First things first - preheat your oven to 225°F (107°C). Yes, it's super low - we're drying these babies out, not baking them!

2. Line a small baking sheet with parchment paper. Don't use wax paper - trust me on this one.

3. In your squeaky-clean bowl, combine the egg white and cream of tartar. Start beating on medium speed until it gets foamy (think bubble bath vibes).

4. Gradually add your sweetener while beating on high speed. Keep going until stiff, glossy peaks form - when you lift the beater, the mixture should stand at attention like a tiny soldier!

5. Here comes the fun part - gently fold in the peppermint extract. Don't go crazy with it unless you want your meringues tasting like toothpaste!

6. Carefully fold in those chocolate chips. Be gentle - we want to keep all that air we just beat in.

7. Transfer the mixture to your piping bag (or zip-top bag with corner snipped).

8. Pipe 6-8 small meringues onto your prepared baking sheet. Go for about 1.5 inches in diameter - they're meant to be bite-sized!

9. Pop them in the oven and let them do their thing for 45-50 minutes. They should be dry to the touch and lift easily from the parchment.

10. Here's the hard part - turn off the oven and LEAVE THEM ALONE for at least 1 hour. I know it's tempting, but don't open that door!

Storage Tips

Store these little delights in an airtight container. They'll keep for about 5 days, if they last that long!

Pro Tips

- Make sure your bowl and beaters are completely free of any grease or egg yolk
- Don't make these on a rainy day (humidity is not your friend)
- If they start to get sticky after storage, pop them in a 200°F oven for 5-10 minutes

Nutritional Information (per meringue, based on 8 servings):

- Calories: 25
- Protein: 0.8g
- Fat: 1.2g
- Net Carbs: 0.5g
- Fiber: 0.3g
- Sugar Alcohols: 2g

Final Note

Remember, these are tiny but mighty! The serving size is 2-3 meringues, which is perfect when you want something sweet but need to stay on track with your Zepbound journey. Plus, they're so light, they practically don't count... (okay, they do count, but they're worth it!)

Chapter 6: Perfectly Portioned Almond Flour Shortbread

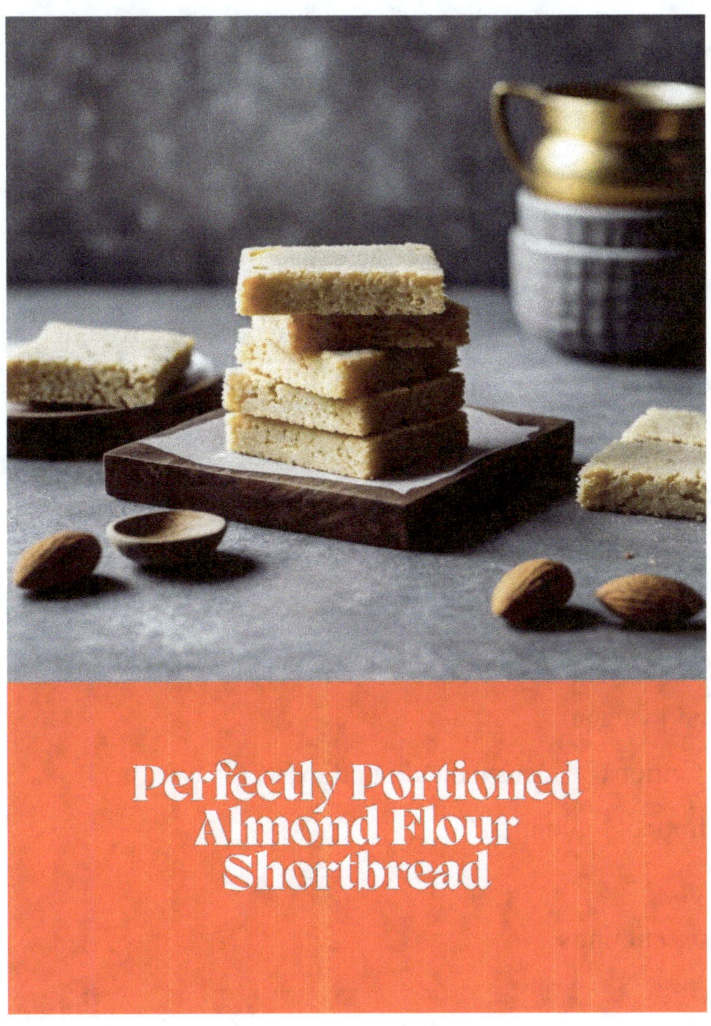

Because sometimes you just need a cookie (or two) without ending up with dozens giving you the side-eye from your kitchen counter

Makes: 4 small cookies (serving size: 1-2 cookies)

Ingredients

- ½ cup blanched almond flour (sifted if you're feeling fancy)
- 2 tablespoons unsalted butter, softened (go ahead, let it lounge on your counter for an hour)
- 1½ tablespoons monk fruit sweetener (or your favorite sugar substitute)
- ¼ teaspoon vanilla extract (the real stuff, because we're worth it)
- Tiny pinch of salt (like, the smallest pinch your fingers can manage)
- Optional: ¼ teaspoon almond extract (for extra almond-y goodness)

Instructions

1. First things first - preheat your oven to 325°F (165°C). Line a small baking sheet with parchment paper. If you're using aluminum foil because you're out of parchment (been there!), give it a light spray with cooking oil.

2. In a small bowl, cream together your softened butter and monk fruit sweetener until it's light and fluffy. This should take about 2 minutes with a fork or spatula. Show those arm muscles who's boss!

3. Add the vanilla extract (and almond extract if you're using it) and that tiny pinch of salt. Mix until combined.

4. Gradually stir in the almond flour. The dough will be a bit crumbly at first - this is normal! Keep mixing until it comes together into a soft dough. It should hold together when you squeeze it.

5. Divide the dough into 4 equal portions (each about 1 tablespoon). Roll each portion into a ball, then gently flatten to about ¼-inch thickness. If you're feeling

artistic, use a fork to make a criss-cross pattern on top (totally optional, but makes them look fancy!).

6. Place cookies on your prepared baking sheet, leaving a little space between each one (they won't spread much, they're well-behaved cookies).

7. Pop them in the oven for 12-15 minutes, or until the edges are just barely starting to turn golden. They should still be quite pale overall.

8. Here's the hard part - let them cool on the baking sheet for 10 minutes! I know it's tempting, but they're quite delicate when hot. After 10 minutes, transfer to a cooling rack (or just eat them, I won't judge).

Storage Tips

These little gems will keep in an airtight container for up to 5 days, but let's be honest - they've never lasted that long in my house! You can also freeze them for up to a month if you're into meal prepping (or hiding cookies from yourself).

Nutritional Information (per cookie):

- Calories: 70

- Total Fat: 6.5g

- Saturated Fat: 2.5g

- Cholesterol: 10mg

- Sodium: 18mg

- Total Carbohydrates: 2g

- Dietary Fiber: 1g

- Net Carbs: 1g

- Protein: 2g

Pro Tips:

- If your dough is too crumbly, add ¼ teaspoon of water

- If your dough is too sticky, add a teaspoon of almond flour

- For perfectly round cookies, use a small cookie cutter or the rim of a shot glass (hey, we're being resourceful here!)

- Let the cookies cool COMPLETELY before handling - they're like tiny divas and need their moment to set

Remember: These cookies are Zepbound-friendly but still should be enjoyed mindfully. They're like tiny hugs for your taste buds, but we don't want to get too huggy, if you know what I mean!

Chapter 7: Protein Sugar Cookies

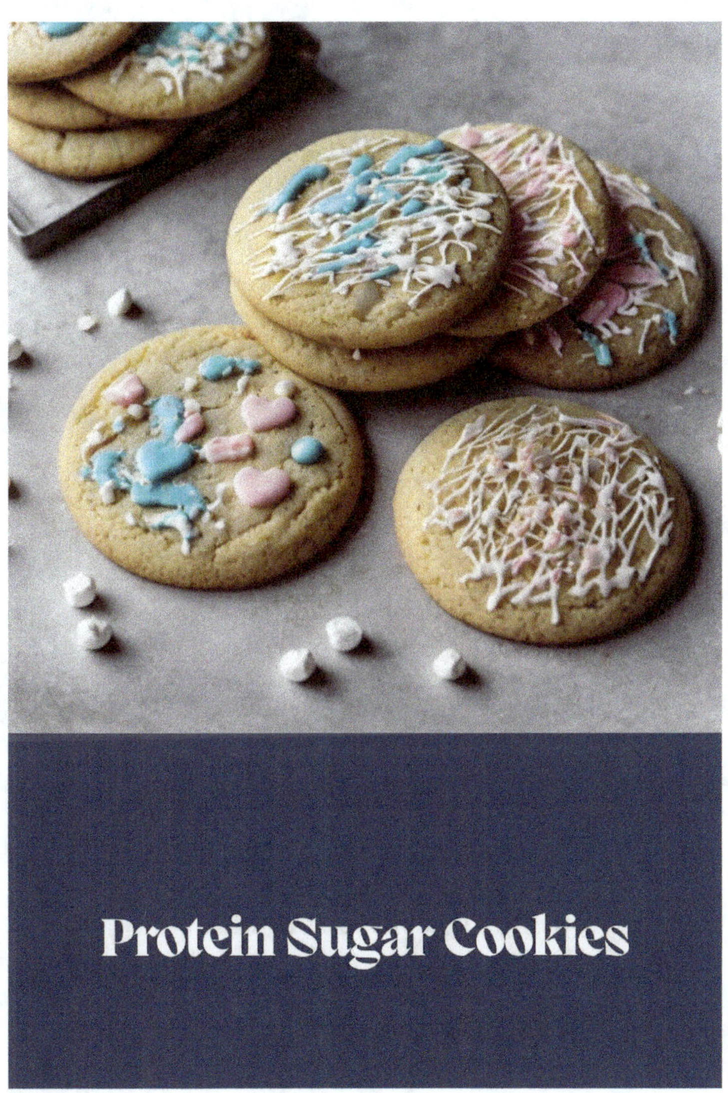

Protein Sugar Cookies

Because who says you can't have cookies while on Zepbound? These adorable little bites of joy will keep both your sweet tooth and your medication happy!

Makes: 2 cookies (perfect for portion control!)

Ingredients

- 2 tablespoons (15g) vanilla whey protein powder
- 1 tablespoon (7g) coconut flour
- 1 tablespoon monk fruit sweetener
- ¼ teaspoon baking powder
- Tiny pinch of salt (just a whisper!)
- 1 tablespoon unsweetened almond milk
- ½ tablespoon melted coconut oil
- ¼ teaspoon vanilla extract
- 1-2 drops natural food coloring (optional, but hey, it's Christmas!)

For the Optional Sugar-Free Sparkle

- ½ teaspoon monk fruit sweetener mixed with a teensy bit of natural food coloring

Instructions

1. Preheat your oven to 350°F (175°C). Line a small baking sheet with parchment paper. (Yes, even for just two cookies - we're fancy like that!)

2. In a small bowl, whisk together your dry ingredients: protein powder, coconut flour, monk fruit sweetener, baking powder, and that whisper of salt. Break up any lumps - we don't want protein powder chunks surprising anyone!

3. In another bowl (or the same one if you're feeling rebellious), mix your wet ingredients: almond milk, melted coconut oil, and vanilla extract. If you're feeling festive, add your food coloring now.

4. Combine wet and dry ingredients until you get a soft dough. If it's too sticky, add a tiny bit more coconut flour. If it's too dry, add a few drops of almond milk. The texture should be similar to Play-Doh (but please don't eat Play-Doh, stick to these cookies instead!)

5. Divide the dough into two equal portions and roll into balls. Place them on your prepared baking sheet and gently press down with a fork to create that classic cookie criss-cross pattern. If you're using the sugar-free sparkle, sprinkle it on now!

6. Bake for 8-10 minutes. The edges should be just slightly firm but not brown. Remember, these are tiny cookies - they bake quickly!

7. Let cool on the baking sheet for 5 minutes (I know it's hard to wait, but your fingers will thank you), then transfer to a cooling rack.

Pro Tips

- Store in an airtight container... though let's be real, they probably won't last that long!
- Feel free to eat both cookies - that's why we made just two!
- Want to make them extra festive? Use green food coloring and shape them like little Christmas trees!

Nutritional Information (per cookie)

- Calories: 45

- Protein: 4g

- Net Carbs: 2g

- Fat: 3g

- Fiber: 1g

- Sugar: 0g

- Guilt: Absolutely none!

Remember: The best cookie is the one you can enjoy without stress. These little gems are designed to let you participate in holiday joy while staying on track with your health goals. Now go forth and bake!

Chapter 8: Chocolate Almond Mini-Batch Biscotti

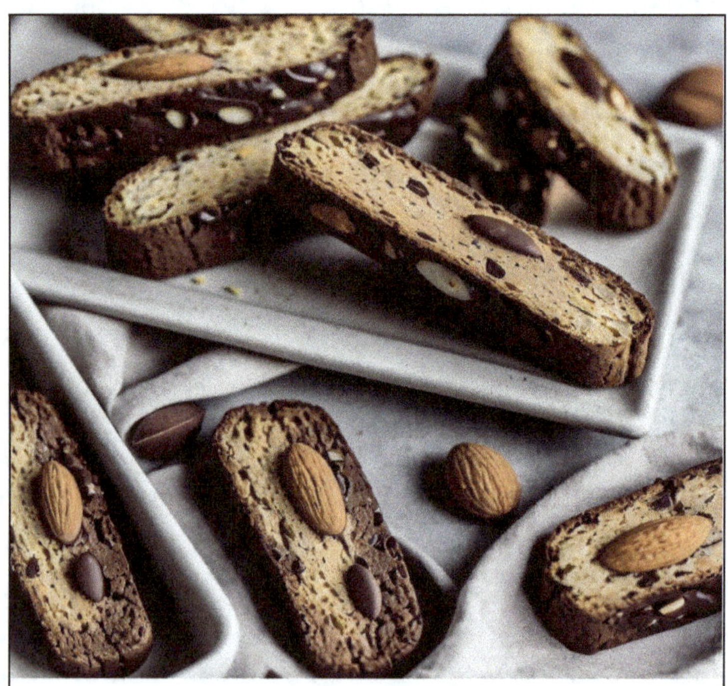

Chocolate Almond Mini–Batch Biscotti

Perfect for when you want that fancy café feeling at home!

Ingredients

(Makes 4-6 biscotti - enough for you and maybe someone you really like)

<u>Dry Ingredients</u>

- 1 cup almond flour (because we're fancy like that)
- 2 tablespoons coconut flour (just enough to make things interesting)
- 2 tablespoons monk fruit sweetener (keeping it Zepbound-friendly!)
- 1 teaspoon baking powder
- ¼ teaspoon salt
- ¼ cup chopped almonds (extra points for toasting them first!)
- 2 tablespoons sugar-free chocolate chips (the tiny ones work best)

<u>Wet Ingredients</u>

- 1 large egg (room temperature, because it deserves comfort too)
- ½ teaspoon vanilla extract
- ¼ teaspoon almond extract (the secret weapon!)

Instructions

<u>First Bake (The Warm-Up Round)</u>

1. Preheat your oven to 350°F (175°C). Line a small baking sheet with parchment paper. (No one likes cleanup duty!)

2. In a medium bowl, whisk together all dry ingredients EXCEPT the chocolate chips and almonds. Think of it as building suspense - they'll join the party later.

3. In a small bowl, beat the egg and extracts until they're well combined and feeling friendly with each other.

4. Pour the wet ingredients into the dry ingredients. Mix until you have a slightly sticky dough. (If it's too wet,

add a tiny bit more coconut flour - like, really tiny, this flour is thirsty!)

5. Now invite the chocolate chips and almonds to the bowl. Fold them in gently - we're not savages here!

6. Shape the dough into a small log on your parchment paper, about 8 inches long and 2 inches wide. (Pro tip: wet hands make this WAY easier)

7. Bake for 20-25 minutes until lightly golden and firm to the touch.

<u>The Cool-Down & Second Bake (Where the Magic Happens)</u>
1. Let your log cool for 15 minutes. (Perfect time to make coffee or scroll through your phone!)

2. Reduce oven temperature to 300°F (150°C).

3. Using a sharp knife (serrated works best), slice the log diagonally into 4-6 pieces, about ½ inch thick each.

4. Lay the slices flat on the baking sheet and bake again for 10-12 minutes on each side until they're nice and crispy. (This is what gives biscotti that satisfying crunch!)

Storage

Store in an airtight container for up to a week, if they last that long!

Serving Suggestions

- Dunk in your morning coffee (I won't judge if it's afternoon coffee)
- Pair with sugar-free hot chocolate
- Enjoy with a cup of tea while pretending you're in a fancy Italian café

Nutritional Information (per biscotti, based on 6 pieces):

- Calories: 60
- Protein: 3g
- Net Carbs: 2g

- Fat: 5g

- Fiber: 2g

- Sugar Alcohols: 1g

Chef's Notes

- If the dough seems too crumbly, add 1 teaspoon of water at a time until it comes together
- For extra pizzazz, drizzle cooled biscotti with melted sugar-free chocolate
- Want to feel extra fancy? Sprinkle with a few sea salt flakes before the first bake

Remember: These aren't Grandma's biscotti - they're your new favorite guilt-free treat that won't have your Zepbound giving you the side-eye!

Chapter 9: Guilt-Free Coconut Macaroons

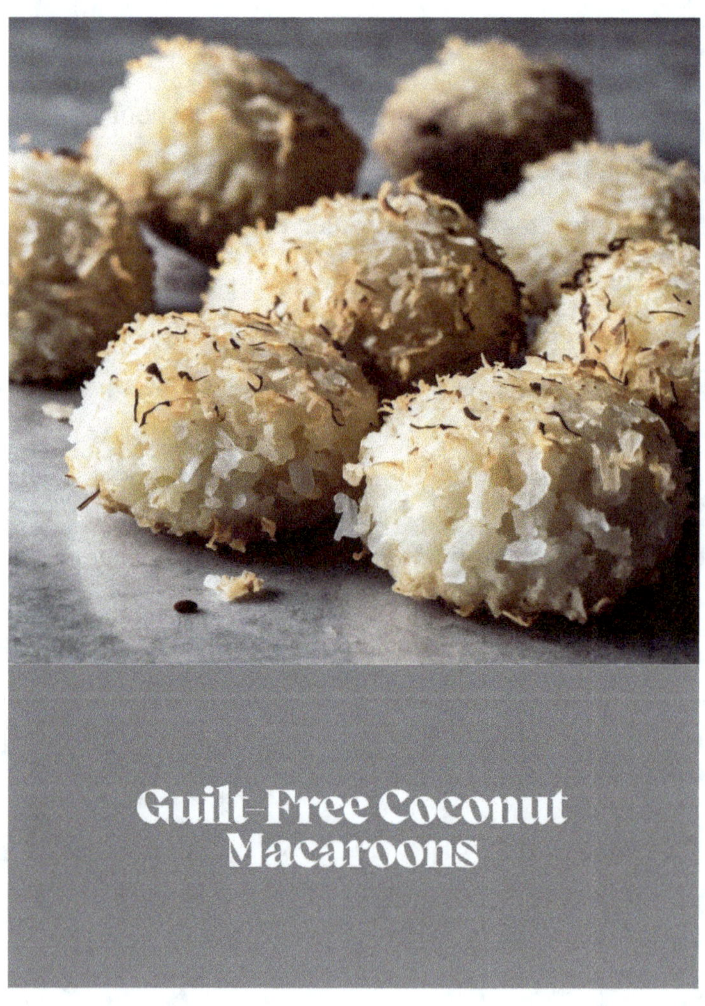

You know that moment when you're staring at a cookie platter like it's your arch-nemesis? Well, these macaroons are here to be your holiday BFF! Let's make just enough for you to enjoy without having a staring contest with a full cookie jar.

Makes: 4 macaroons (perfect for 2 servings or 2 days of treats!)

What You'll Need:

- 1 cup unsweetened shredded coconut (the hero of our story!)

- 1 large egg white (just one lonely soldier doing its duty)

- 2 tablespoons monk fruit sweetener (because we're sweet enough already)

- ¼ teaspoon vanilla extract (the little flavor that could!)

- Tiny pinch of salt (just a hello's worth)

- Optional: 1 tablespoon sugar-free chocolate chips for drizzling (because sometimes we need to live a little!)

The Magic Steps:

1. Preheat your oven to 325°F (or 165°C if you're fancy and European)

2. Line a small baking sheet with parchment paper (no cookie left behind!)

3. In a bowl, whisk that egg white until it's frothy and full of itself (about 30 seconds)

4. Toss in your monk fruit sweetener, vanilla, and that friendly pinch of salt. Give it another whisk until it's looking glossy and proud.

5. Fold in your coconut until it's all coated. (Think of it as giving each coconut shred a tiny hug)

6. Using slightly wet hands (trust me on this!), form 4 compact balls about 1½ inches each. Place them on your prepared baking sheet like little soldiers.

7. Bake for 15-18 minutes or until they're golden brown on the edges. (Watch them like a helicopter parent - they can go from perfect to "oops" pretty quick!)

8. Let them cool completely on the baking sheet (patience is a virtue, my friend!)

<u>Optional Fancy Pants Step:</u>
If you're feeling extra, melt those sugar-free chocolate chips in the microwave (30 seconds, stir, repeat if needed) and drizzle over the cooled macaroons like you're Jackson Pollock.

Nutritional Breakdown (Per Macaroon):
- Calories: 45
- Protein: 1g
- Fat: 4g
- Net Carbs: 1g
- Fiber: 1g
- Sugar: 0g
- Guilt: Absolutely zero!

Storage Wisdom:

Store these little beauties in an airtight container for up to 3 days... though let's be real, they rarely last that long!

Pro Tip:

If you're having a "I could eat all of these" moment, remember that freezing them works great! They'll last up to a month frozen, and they taste amazing straight from the freezer. It's like portion control with a built-in waiting period - genius, right?

Remember: Living your best Zepbound life doesn't mean saying goodbye to cookies - it just means saying hello to smarter, yummier choices! These macaroons are so good, you might catch your non-dieting friends trying to steal them. Guard them wisely!

Now go forth and conquer those holiday cravings, you magnificent cookie warrior!

Chapter 10: Pecan Sandies

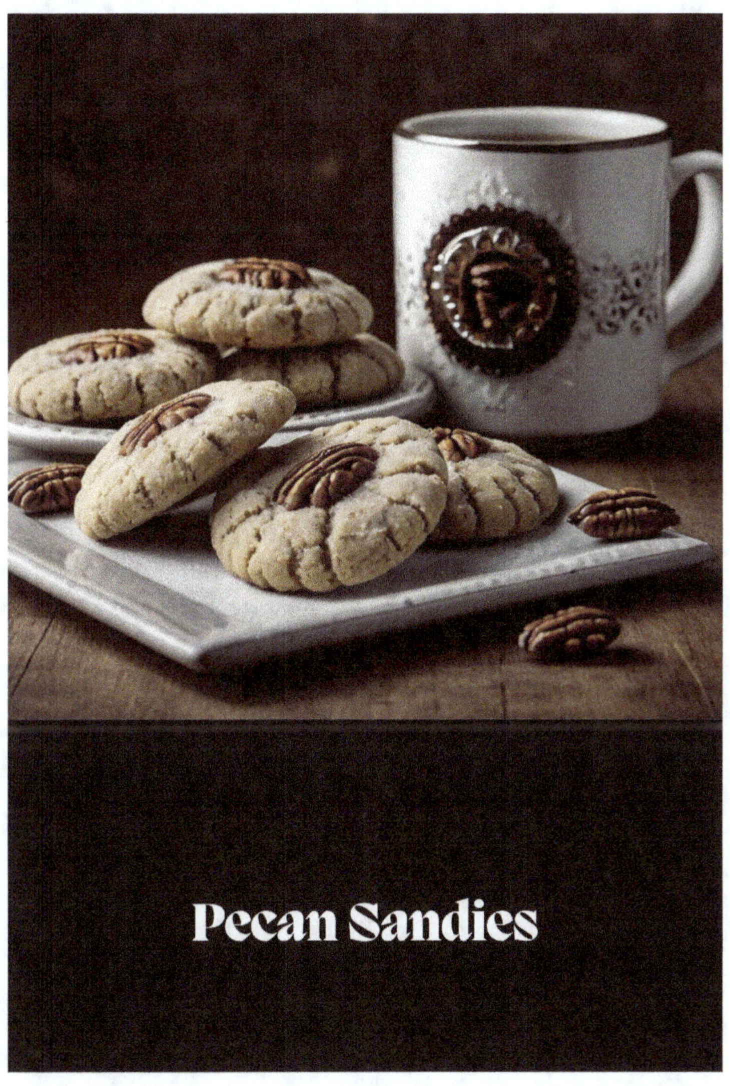

Oh boy, do I have the perfect recipe for you! These Pecan Sandies are a classic holiday cookie with a delightful twist. Get ready to impress your friends and family with these nutty, buttery delights.

Ingredients:
- 1 cup (120g) almond flour
- 1/2 cup (50g) chopped pecans
- 1/4 cup (50g) monk fruit sweetener
- 1 teaspoon vanilla extract
- 1/4 teaspoon salt

Instructions:
1. Preheat your oven to a toasty 350°F (175°C). Line a baking sheet with parchment paper - we want these cookies to slide right off when they're done!

2. In a food processor, give those pecans a whirl until they're finely chopped. Now add the almond flour, monk fruit sweetener, vanilla, and salt. Pulse until the mixture

starts to come together in a soft dough. If it's a little dry, add a teaspoon of water and give it another quick pulse.

3. Scoop the dough by the tablespoonful and roll it into 1-inch balls. Arrange them on the prepared baking sheet, leaving a bit of space between each one. These little guys are going to spread out a bit as they bake.

4. Pop the tray in the oven and let the magic happen for 12-15 minutes. Keep an eye on them - you want the edges to be lightly golden and the centers still a touch soft.

5. Once they're out of the oven, let the cookies cool on the baking sheet for 5 minutes before transferring them to a wire rack. This helps them hold their shape.

These Pecan Sandies are the perfect balance of nutty, buttery, and just a touch sweet. Pair them with a hot cup of coffee or tea for the ultimate cozy holiday treat. Plus, they're Zepbound-friendly, so you can indulge without the guilt!

Nutritional Info (per cookie):

Calories: 65

Fat: 5g

Carbs: 5g

Protein: 2g

Enjoy, my friend! And remember, life's too short for boring cookies. These Pecan Sandies are here to add a little joy to your day.

Chapter 11: Cream Cheese Sugar Cookies

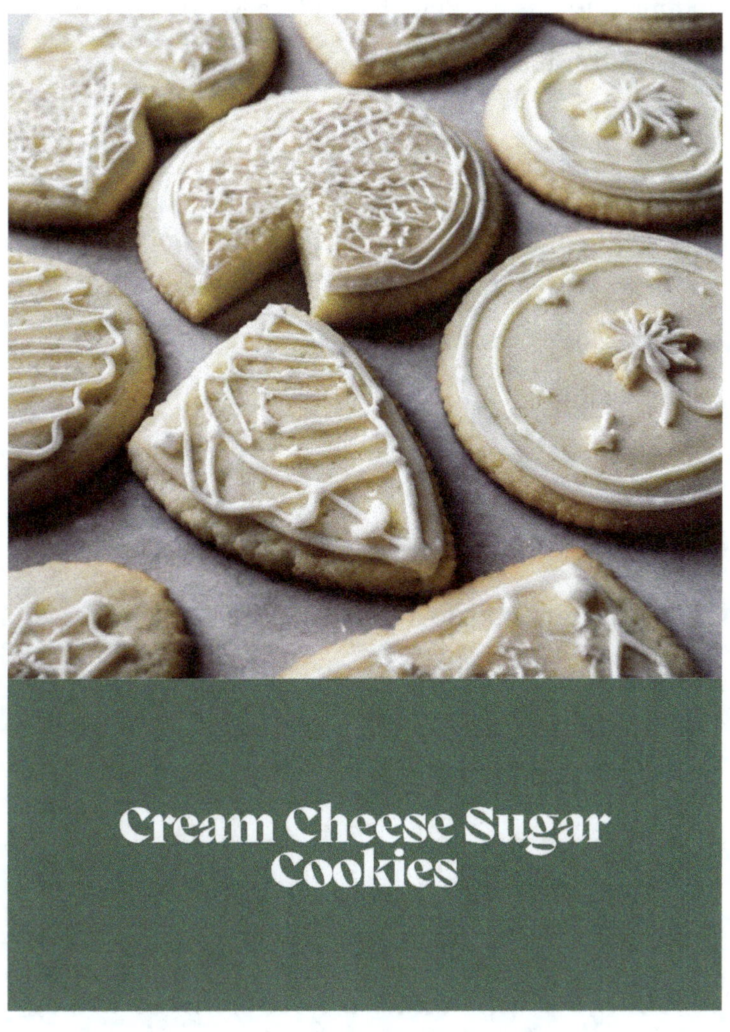

Ah, the Cream Cheese Sugar Cookies - a delightful little morsel that'll have your taste buds dancing the jig! These pillowy soft treats are the perfect balance of indulgence and mindfulness, making them a true MVP in the Zepbound-friendly cookie lineup.

Ingredients:

- 2 oz low-fat cream cheese, softened
- 1/4 cup almond flour
- 2 tbsp Monk fruit sweetener
- 1 tsp vanilla extract
- Pinch of salt

Instructions:

1. Preheat your oven to a toasty 350°F (175°C). Line a baking sheet with parchment paper, because we all know how those pesky cookies can get a bit clingy if we don't give them a helping hand.

2. In a mixing bowl fit for a baking champion, combine the softened cream cheese, almond flour, Monk fruit sweetener, vanilla extract, and a wee pinch of salt. Mix

until the dough comes together in a delightful, pliable ball. Don't be afraid to get in there with your hands - it's the only way to truly become one with the cookie dough!

3. Scoop out the dough by the heaping tablespoonful and roll them into cute little rounds, about 1-inch in diameter. Arrange these precious gems on your prepared baking sheet, making sure to leave a smidge of space between each one - we don't want any cookie casualties!

4. Pop that tray into the oven and let the magic happen. Bake for 10-12 minutes, or until the edges are ever-so-slightly golden and the centers are still soft and pillowy. It's like they're giving you a little hug with every bite.

5. Once they've had their time in the oven, remove the tray and let the cookies cool completely on the sheet. This allows the centers to firm up just a touch, but still maintain that irresistible, melt-in-your-mouth texture.

Serving Size: 1-2 cookies

Nutritional Information (per 1 cookie):

- Calories: 50

- Total Fat: 3g

- Carbohydrates: 4g

- Protein: 2g

- Fiber: 1g

- Sugar: 2g

Go ahead, treat yourself to one (or two!) of these little delights. They're the perfect way to satisfy that sweet tooth while keeping your Zepbound journey on track. Enjoy, my fellow cookie connoisseurs!

Chapter 12: Chocolate Mint Wafers

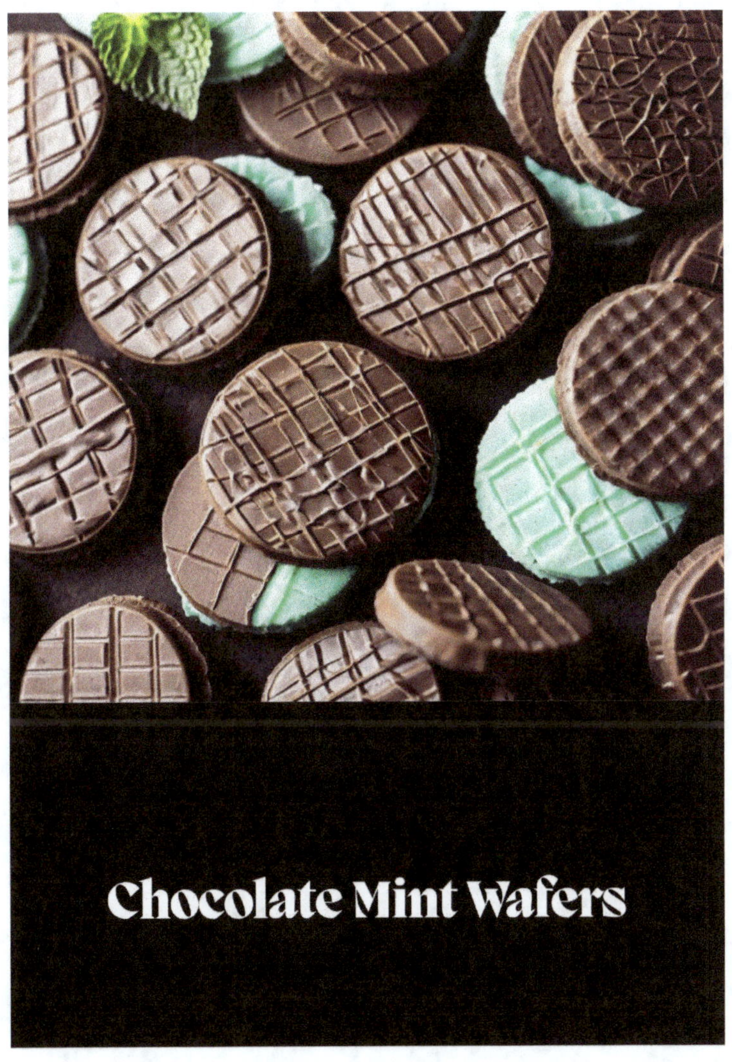

Ooh, the Chocolate Mint Wafers - now we're talking! These delightful little discs of chocolatey goodness are like a breath of fresh (sugar-free) air in the cookie realm. Grab your mixing bowls and let's get baking, my friends!

Ingredients:
- 1/2 cup coconut flour
- 2 tbsp unsweetened cocoa powder
- 1 tsp peppermint extract
- 2 tbsp Monk fruit sweetener
- Pinch of salt
- 2 tbsp sugar-free chocolate chips (for topping)

Instructions:
1. Preheat your oven to a toasty 350°F (175°C) and line a baking sheet with parchment paper, because we all know how those pesky cookies can get a bit clingy if we don't give them a helping hand.

2. In a mixing bowl fit for a baking champion, combine the coconut flour, unsweetened cocoa powder, peppermint extract, Monk fruit sweetener, and a pinch of

salt. Mix it all together until it forms a delightfully fudgy dough. It's like a minty chocolate dream come true!

3. Scoop out the dough by the heaping tablespoonful and roll them into cute little discs, about 1-inch in diameter. Arrange these precious gems on your prepared baking sheet, making sure to leave a smidge of space between each one - we don't want any cookie casualties!

4. Top each cookie with a few sugar-free chocolate chips, because who doesn't love a little extra chocolatey goodness?

5. Pop that tray into the oven and let the magic happen. Bake for 8-10 minutes, or until the edges are just starting to crisp up and the centers are still delightfully soft and fudgy. It's like a little chocolate-mint explosion in your mouth!

6. Once they've had their time in the oven, remove the tray and let the cookies cool completely on the sheet.

This allows the centers to firm up just a touch, but still maintain that irresistible, melt-in-your-mouth texture.

Serving Size: 1-2 cookies

Nutritional Information (per 1 cookie):
- Calories: 40
- Total Fat: 2g
- Carbohydrates: 6g
- Protein: 1g
- Fiber: 2g
- Sugar: 1g

Chapter 13: Peanut Butter Blossoms

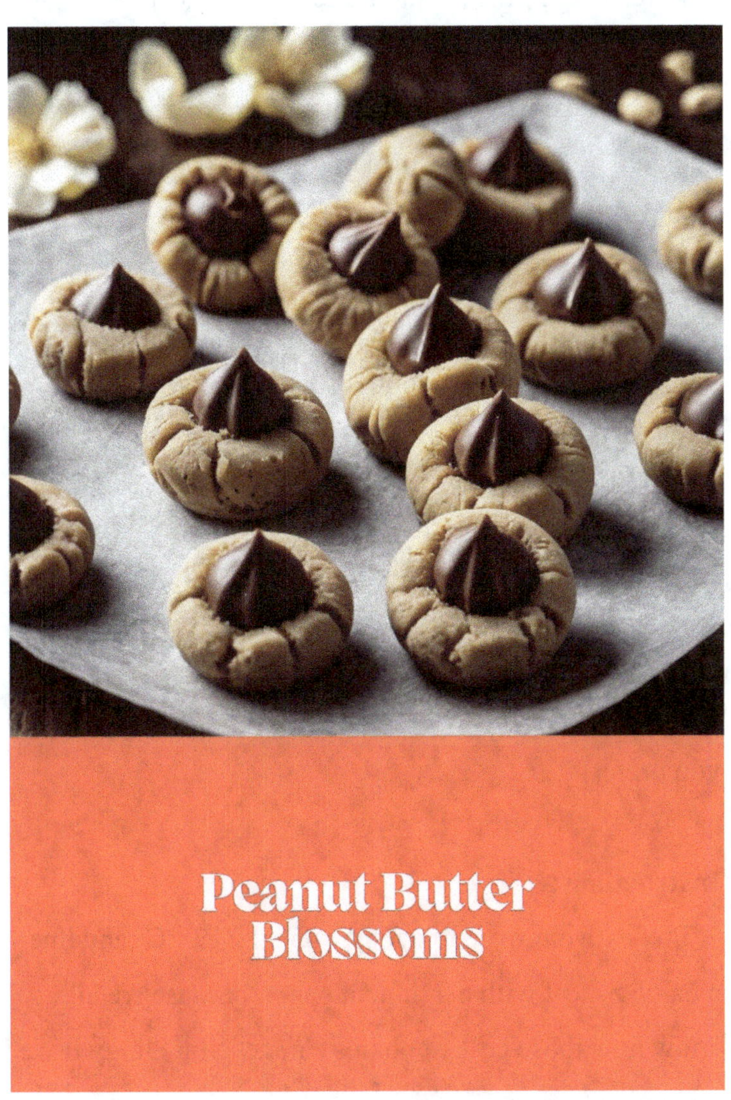

Ah, the Peanut Butter Blossoms - now we're really talking! These little peanut butter delights with a sugar-free chocolate kiss on top are about to become your new best friends. Gather your ingredients and let's get ready to bake up a storm, my fellow cookie enthusiasts.

Ingredients:

- 1/4 cup natural peanut butter (the kind that makes you wanna lick the spoon)
- 2 tbsp vanilla protein powder
- 1 tbsp Monk fruit sweetener
- 1 tsp vanilla extract
- Pinch of salt
- 12 sugar-free chocolate kisses (or chocolate chips if you prefer)

Instructions:

1. Preheat your oven to a toasty 350°F (175°C) and line a baking sheet with parchment paper, because we all know how those pesky cookies can get a bit clingy if we don't give them a helping hand.

2. In a mixing bowl fit for a baking champion, combine the natural peanut butter, vanilla protein powder, Monk fruit sweetener, vanilla extract, and a pinch of salt. Mix it all together until it forms a delightfully smooth and creamy dough. It's like a peanut butter dream come true!

3. Scoop out the dough by the heaping tablespoonful and roll them into cute little rounds, about 1-inch in diameter. Arrange these precious gems on your prepared baking sheet, making sure to leave a smidge of space between each one - we don't want any cookie casualties!

4. Gently press a sugar-free chocolate kiss (or a few chocolate chips) into the center of each cookie, because who doesn't love a little extra chocolatey goodness?

5. Pop that tray into the oven and let the magic happen. Bake for 8-10 minutes, or until the edges are just starting to turn a lovely golden brown and the centers are still delightfully soft and peanut buttery. It's like a little taste of heaven in every bite!

6. Once they've had their time in the oven, remove the tray and let the cookies cool completely on the sheet. This allows the centers to firm up just a touch, but still maintain that irresistible, melt-in-your-mouth texture.

Serving Size: 1-2 cookies

Nutritional Information (per 1 cookie):
- Calories: 75
- Total Fat: 5g
- Carbohydrates: 5g
- Protein: 3g
- Fiber: 1g
- Sugar: 2g

Chapter 14: Cranberry Almond Cookies

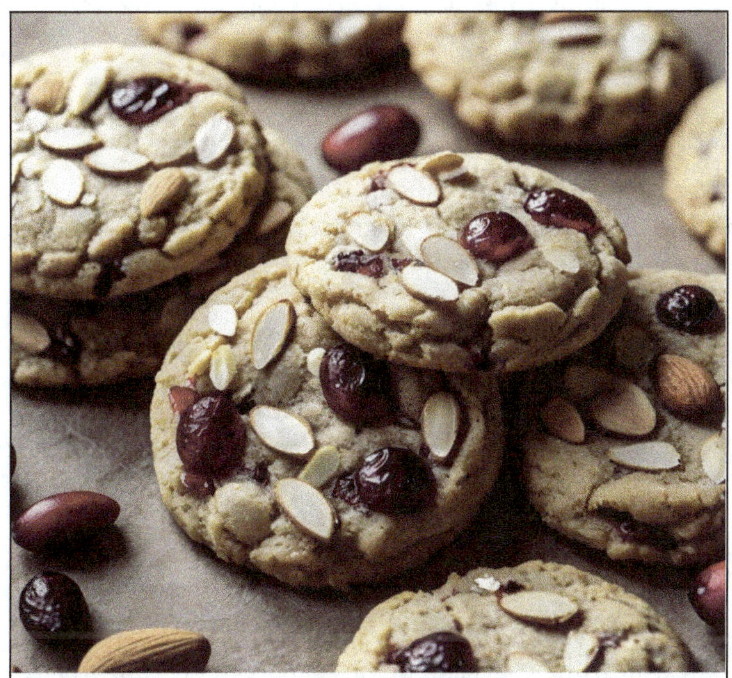

Ingredients:

- 1 cup almond flour (because who doesn't love a little nutty goodness?)
- 2 tbsp Monk fruit sweetener (to keep things nice and low-sugar)
- 1/4 cup sugar-free dried cranberries (tart and tangy, just how we like it!)
- 2 tbsp sliced almonds (for that extra crunch factor)
- 1 tsp vanilla extract (because vanilla makes everything better)
- Pinch of salt (to balance out all that sweetness)

Instructions:

1. Preheat your oven to a toasty 350°F (175°C) and line a baking sheet with parchment paper, because we all know how those pesky cookies can get a bit clingy if we don't give them a helping hand.

2. In a mixing bowl fit for a baking champion, combine the almond flour, Monk fruit sweetener, sugar-free dried cranberries, sliced almonds, vanilla extract, and a pinch

of salt. Mix it all together until it forms a delightfully textured dough. It's like a flavor party waiting to happen!

3. Scoop out the dough by the heaping tablespoonful and roll them into cute little rounds, about 1-inch in diameter. Arrange these precious gems on your prepared baking sheet, making sure to leave a smidge of space between each one - we don't want any cookie casualties!

4. Pop that tray into the oven and let the magic happen. Bake for 10-12 minutes, or until the edges are ever-so-slightly golden and the centers are still soft and chewy. It's like a little taste of winter wonderland in every bite!

5. Once they've had their time in the oven, remove the tray and let the cookies cool completely on the sheet. This allows the centers to firm up just a touch, but still maintain that irresistible, melt-in-your-mouth texture.

Serving Size: 1-2 cookies

Nutritional Information (per 1 cookie):

- Calories: 60

- Total Fat: 4g

- Carbohydrates: 6g

- Protein: 2g

- Fiber: 2g

- Sugar: 2g

Chapter 15: Lemon Ricotta Cookies

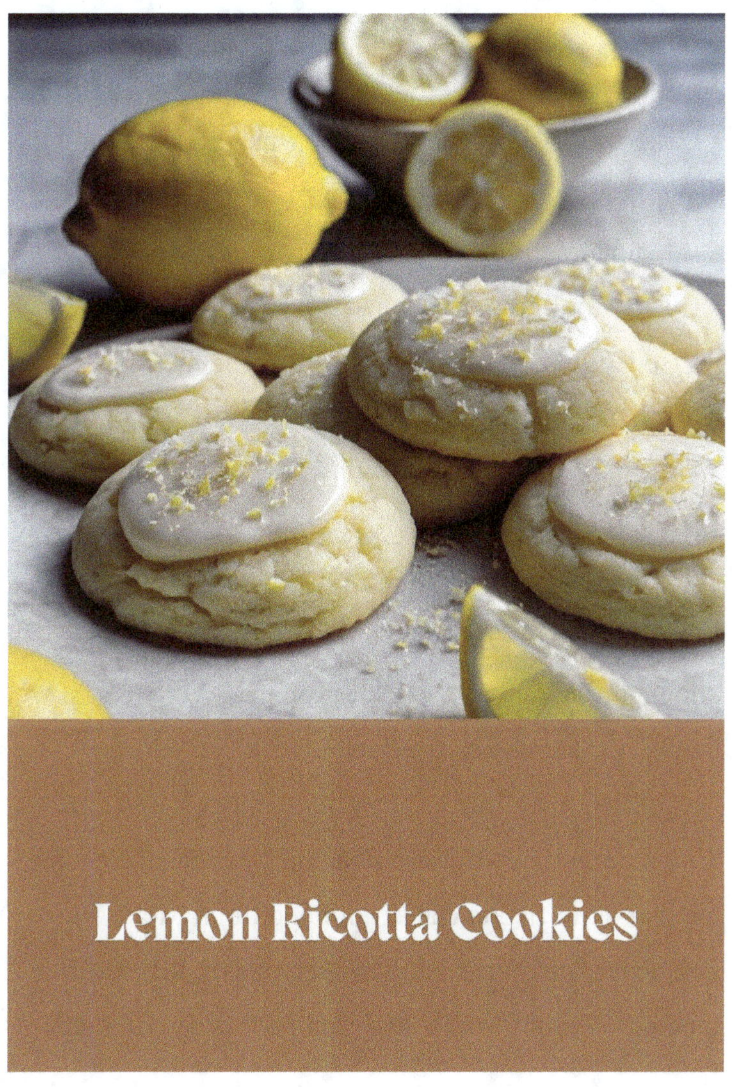

Ahh, the Lemon Ricotta Cookies - a little slice of sunshine in cookie form!

Ingredients:

- 1/2 cup part-skim ricotta cheese (the good stuff, not the watery kind)
- 1/4 cup almond flour
- 1 tbsp Monk fruit sweetener
- 1 tsp lemon zest (trust me, the more the merrier)
- Pinch of salt

Instructions:

1. Preheat your oven to a toasty 350°F (175°C) and line a baking sheet with parchment paper, because we all know how those pesky cookies can get a bit clingy if we don't give them a helping hand.

2. In a mixing bowl fit for a baking champion, combine the part-skim ricotta cheese, almond flour, Monk fruit sweetener, lemon zest, and a pinch of salt. Mix it all together until it forms a delightfully creamy and tangy

dough. It's like a party in your mouth, just waiting to happen!

3. Scoop out the dough by the heaping tablespoonful and roll them into cute little rounds, about 1-inch in diameter. Arrange these precious gems on your prepared baking sheet, making sure to leave a smidge of space between each one - we don't want any cookie casualties!

4. Pop that tray into the oven and let the magic happen. Bake for 10-12 minutes, or until the edges are just starting to turn a lovely golden brown and the centers are still delightfully soft and pillowy. It's like a little lemon-infused hug in every bite!

5. Once they've had their time in the oven, remove the tray and let the cookies cool completely on the sheet. This allows the centers to firm up just a touch, but still maintain that irresistible, melt-in-your-mouth texture.

Serving Size: 1-2 cookies

Nutritional Information (per 1 cookie):

- Calories: 55

- Total Fat: 2g

- Carbohydrates: 6g

- Protein: 3g

- Fiber: 1g

- Sugar: 2g

Chapter 16: Spiced Chai Cookies

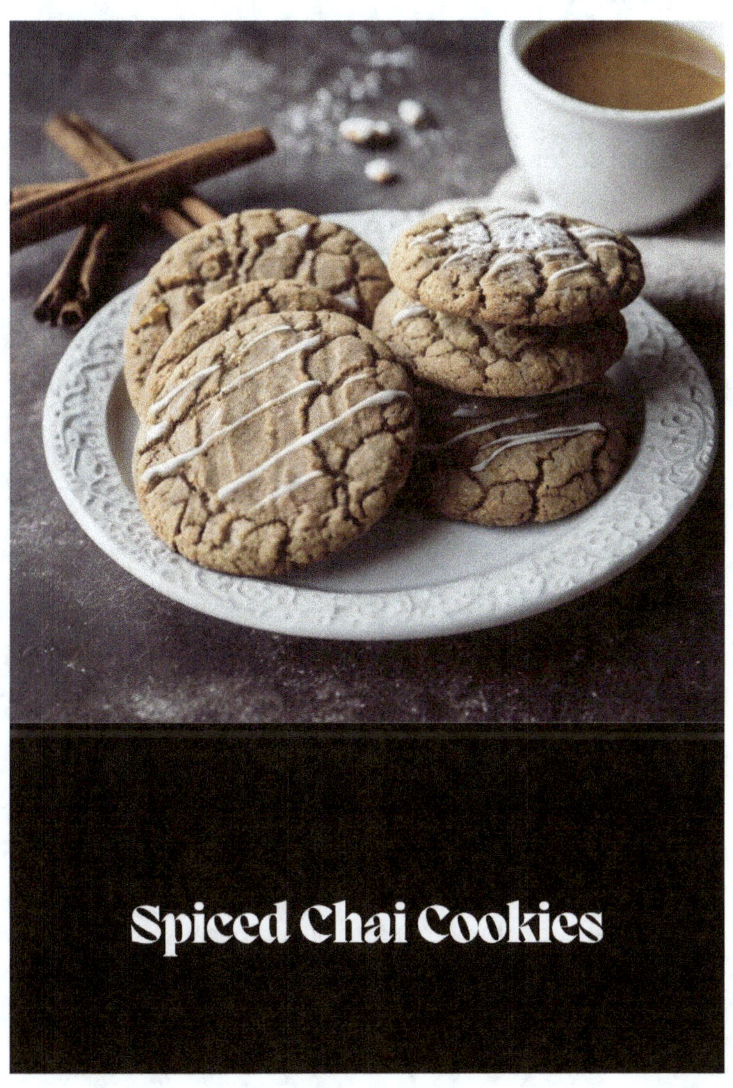

These fragrant little morsels are like a warm hug in cookie form.

Ingredients:
- 1/2 cup coconut flour (the secret to fluffy, cloud-like cookies)
- 1 tsp ground cinnamon
- 1/2 tsp ground cardamom
- 1/4 tsp ground ginger
- 1/4 tsp ground cloves
- 2 tbsp Monk fruit sweetener (because we're keeping things Zepbound-friendly, of course)
- 1 tbsp vanilla protein powder (for an extra boost of protein power)
- Pinch of salt

Instructions:
1. Preheat your oven to a toasty 350°F (175°C) and line a baking sheet with parchment paper, because we all know how those pesky cookies can get a bit clingy if we don't give them a helping hand.

2. In a mixing bowl fit for a baking champion, combine the coconut flour, ground cinnamon, cardamom, ginger, cloves, Monk fruit sweetener, vanilla protein powder, and a pinch of salt. Mix it all together until it forms a delightfully fragrant and spicy dough. It's like a little chai tea party in your mouth!

3. Scoop out the dough by the heaping tablespoonful and roll them into cute little rounds, about 1-inch in diameter. Arrange these precious gems on your prepared baking sheet, making sure to leave a smidge of space between each one - we don't want any cookie casualties!

4. Pop that tray into the oven and let the magic happen. Bake for 10-12 minutes, or until the edges are just starting to turn a lovely golden brown and the centers are still delightfully soft and spicy. It's like a little taste of chai heaven in every bite!

5. Once they've had their time in the oven, remove the tray and let the cookies cool completely on the sheet.

This allows the centers to firm up just a touch, but still maintain that irresistible, melt-in-your-mouth texture.

Serving Size: 1-2 cookies

Nutritional Information (per 1 cookie):
- Calories: 45
- Total Fat: 2g
- Carbohydrates: 5g
- Protein: 2g
- Fiber: 2g
- Sugar: 1g

Chapter 17: Orange-Cardamom Shortbread

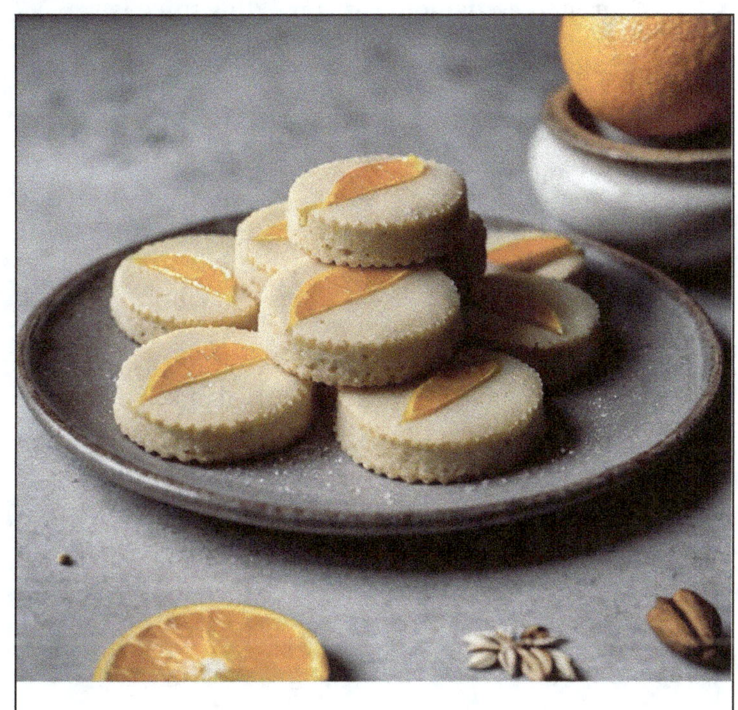

Ingredients:

- 1/2 cup almond flour (the secret to shortbread success!)
- 1 tsp orange zest (the more the merrier, I say!)
- 1/2 tsp ground cardamom (trust me, this spice is a game-changer)
- 2 tbsp Monk fruit sweetener (because we're keeping things Zepbound-friendly, of course)
- Pinch of salt (to really make those flavors pop)

Instructions:

1. Preheat your oven to a toasty 350°F (175°C) and line a baking sheet with parchment paper, because we all know how those pesky cookies can get a bit clingy if we don't give them a helping hand.

2. In a mixing bowl fit for a baking champion, combine the almond flour, orange zest, ground cardamom, Monk fruit sweetener, and a pinch of salt. Mix it all together until it forms a delightfully crumbly and aromatic dough. It's like a flavor explosion just waiting to happen!

3. Scoop out the dough by the heaping tablespoonful and roll them into cute little rounds, about 1-inch in diameter. Arrange these precious gems on your prepared baking sheet, making sure to leave a smidge of space between each one - we don't want any cookie casualties!

4. Pop that tray into the oven and let the magic happen. Bake for 10-12 minutes, or until the edges are just starting to turn a lovely golden brown and the centers are still delightfully soft and tender. It's like a little taste of citrusy, spicy heaven in every bite!

5. Once they've had their time in the oven, remove the tray and let the cookies cool completely on the sheet. This allows the centers to firm up just a touch, but still maintain that irresistible, melt-in-your-mouth texture.

Serving Size: 1-2 cookies

Nutritional Information (per 1 cookie):
- Calories: 65
- Total Fat: 4g

- Carbohydrates: 6g

- Protein: 2g

- Fiber: 1g

- Sugar: 2g

Chapter 18: Chocolate Sandwich Cookies

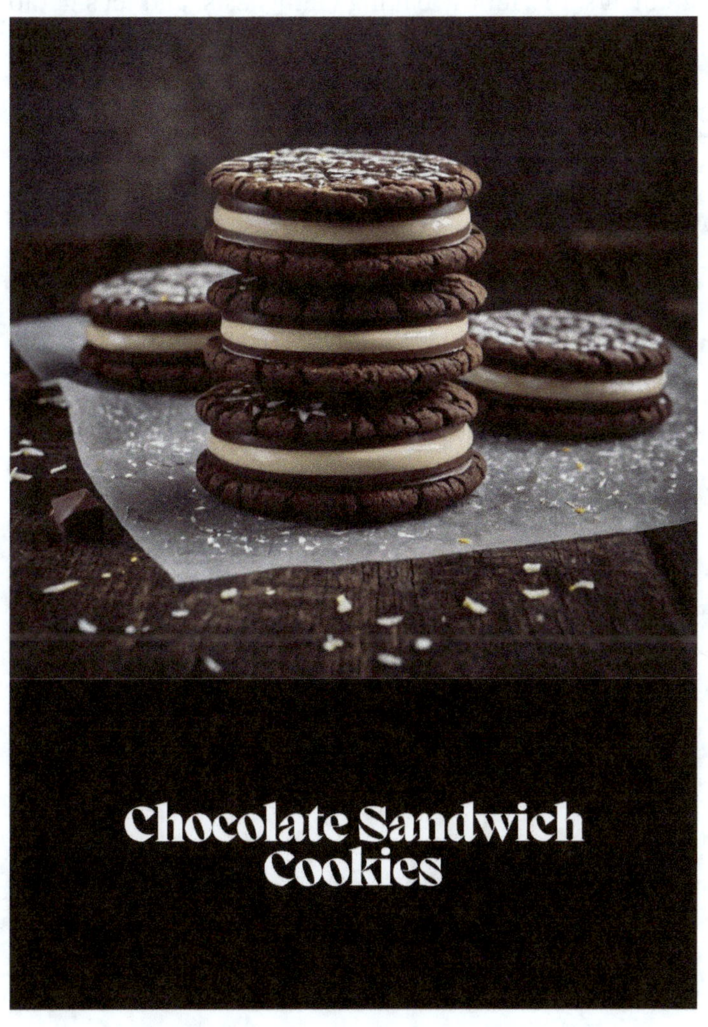

Ah, the Chocolate Sandwich Cookies - now we're talking about a real treat! These little pockets of chocolatey goodness are like a hug for your taste buds. Gather your ingredients, my fellow baking enthusiasts, and let's get to work on creating a cookie sensation that's sure to impress.

Ingredients:

- 1/2 cup cocoa powder (the dark, rich kind that makes your mouth water)
- 1/4 cup almond flour (for that perfect, tender crumb)
- 2 tbsp Monk fruit sweetener (to keep things Zepbound-friendly, of course)
- 1/4 cup sugar-free cream cheese (the secret to that dreamy filling)
- 1 tsp vanilla extract (because every good cookie needs a little vanilla oomph)
- Pinch of salt (to really make those flavors pop)

Instructions:

1. Preheat your oven to a toasty 350°F (175°C) and line a baking sheet with parchment paper, because we all

know how those pesky cookies can get a bit clingy if we don't give them a helping hand.

2. In a mixing bowl fit for a baking champion, combine the cocoa powder, almond flour, and Monk fruit sweetener. Mix it all together until it forms a rich, chocolatey dough. It's like a chocolate lover's dream come true!

3. Scoop out the dough by the heaping tablespoonful and roll them into cute little rounds, about 1-inch in diameter. Arrange these precious gems on your prepared baking sheet, making sure to leave a smidge of space between each one - we don't want any cookie casualties!

4. Pop that tray into the oven and let the magic happen. Bake for 8-10 minutes, or until the edges are just starting to crisp up and the centers are still delightfully soft and fudgy. It's like a little chocolate explosion in every bite!

5. While the cookies are baking, grab a small bowl and whip up the sugar-free cream cheese filling by mixing it

with the vanilla extract and a pinch of salt. Get ready for some serious flavor synergy, folks!

6. Once the cookies have had their time in the oven, remove the tray and let them cool completely on the sheet. This allows the centers to firm up just a touch, but still maintain that irresistible, melt-in-your-mouth texture.

7. Finally, it's time to assemble your masterpiece! Carefully spread a dollop of the creamy filling onto the flat side of one cookie, then top it with another cookie to create a delectable sandwich. Repeat with the remaining cookies and filling.

Serving Size: 1-2 cookies

Nutritional Information (per 1 cookie):
- Calories: 70
- Total Fat: 4g
- Carbohydrates: 7g
- Protein: 2g

- Fiber: 2g
- Sugar: 2g

Chapter 19: Maple Pecan Cookies

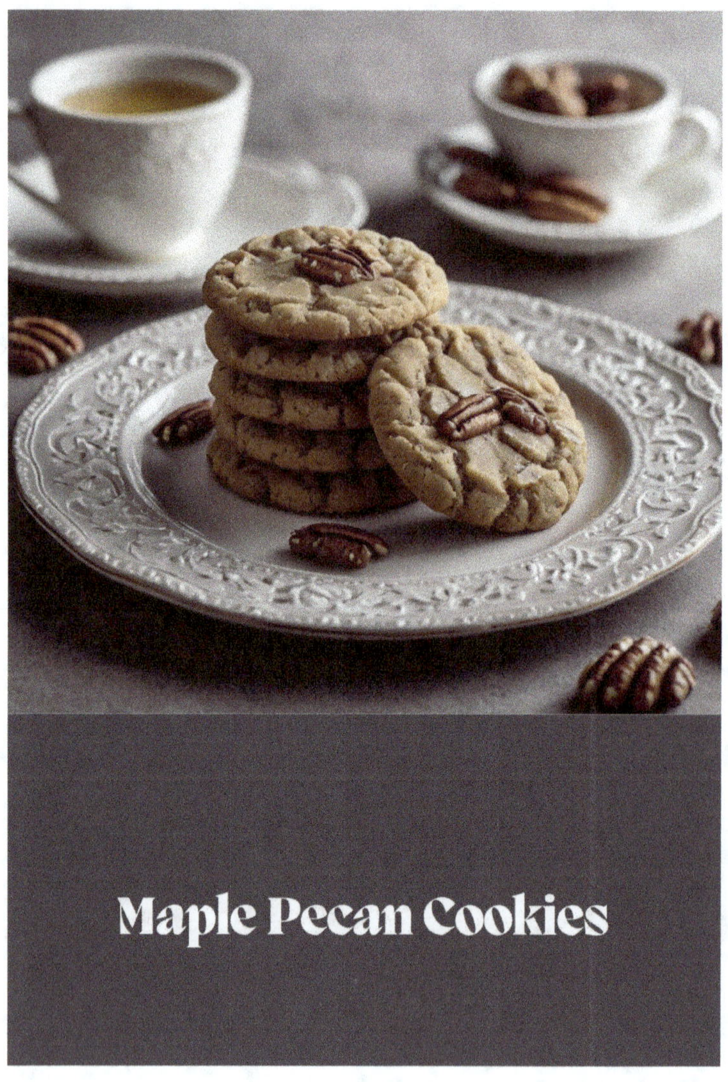

These little nuggets of nutty, maple-y goodness are about to become your new best friends.

Ingredients:

- 1/2 cup pecan flour (because who doesn't love a little nutty flair?)
- 1/4 cup almond flour (for that perfect tender crumb)
- 2 tbsp sugar-free maple syrup (the real deal, not that imitation stuff)
- 1 tbsp Monk fruit sweetener (we're keeping it Zepbound-friendly, my friends)
- 1/2 tsp ground cinnamon (because a little warmth never hurt anyone)
- Pinch of salt (to really make those flavors sing)

Instructions:

1. Preheat your oven to a toasty 350°F (175°C) and line a baking sheet with parchment paper, because we all know how those pesky cookies can get a bit clingy if we don't give them a helping hand.

2. In a mixing bowl fit for a baking champion, combine the pecan flour, almond flour, sugar-free maple syrup, Monk fruit sweetener, ground cinnamon, and a pinch of salt. Mix it all together until it forms a delightfully nutty and aromatic dough. It's like a little taste of the maple syrup-covered forests of Canada, but without all the sugar!

3. Scoop out the dough by the heaping tablespoonful and roll them into cute little rounds, about 1-inch in diameter. Arrange these precious gems on your prepared baking sheet, making sure to leave a smidge of space between each one - we don't want any cookie casualties!

4. Pop that tray into the oven and let the magic happen. Bake for 10-12 minutes, or until the edges are just starting to turn a lovely golden brown and the centers are still delightfully soft and tender. It's like a little hug for your taste buds in every bite!

5. Once they've had their time in the oven, remove the tray and let the cookies cool completely on the sheet.

This allows the centers to firm up just a touch, but still maintain that irresistible, melt-in-your-mouth texture.

Serving Size: 1-2 cookies

Nutritional Information (per 1 cookie):
- Calories: 60
- Total Fat: 4g
- Carbohydrates: 5g
- Protein: 1g
- Fiber: 2g
- Sugar: 2g

Chapter 20: Pistachio Cookies

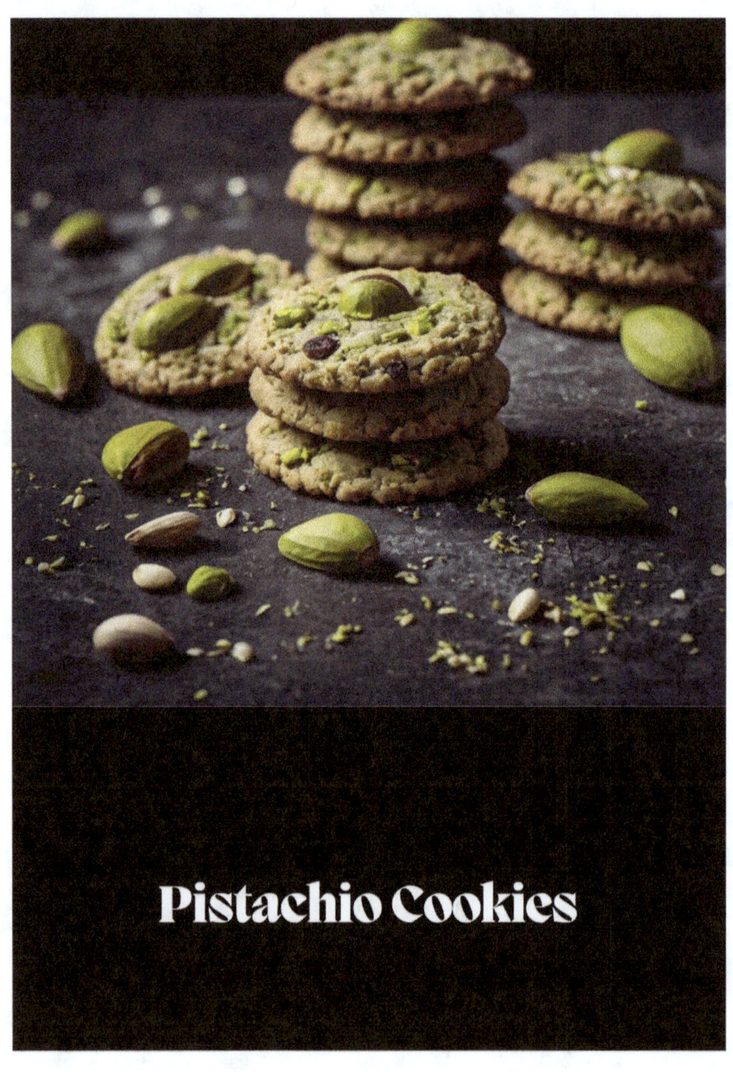

Ingredients:

- 1/2 cup ground pistachios (the secret to these cookies' nutty deliciousness)
- 1/4 cup almond flour (for that perfect tender crumb)
- 2 tbsp Monk fruit sweetener (because we're keeping things low in sugar, my friends)
- 1 tsp almond extract (to really make those nutty flavors pop)
- Pinch of salt (to balance out all that goodness)

Instructions:

1. Preheat your oven to a toasty 350°F (175°C) and line a baking sheet with parchment paper, because we all know how those pesky cookies can get a bit clingy if we don't give them a helping hand.

2. In a mixing bowl fit for a baking champion, combine the ground pistachios, almond flour, Monk fruit sweetener, almond extract, and a pinch of salt. Mix it all together until it forms a delightfully crumbly and fragrant dough. It's like a little pistachio party in your mouth, just waiting to happen!

3. Scoop out the dough by the heaping tablespoonful and roll them into cute little rounds, about 1-inch in diameter. Arrange these precious gems on your prepared baking sheet, making sure to leave a smidge of space between each one - we don't want any cookie casualties!

4. Pop that tray into the oven and let the magic happen. Bake for 10-12 minutes, or until the edges are just starting to turn a lovely golden brown and the centers are still delightfully soft and tender. It's like a little taste of pistachio heaven in every bite!

5. Once they've had their time in the oven, remove the tray and let the cookies cool completely on the sheet. This allows the centers to firm up just a touch, but still maintain that irresistible, melt-in-your-mouth texture.

Serving Size: 1-2 cookies

Nutritional Information (per 1 cookie):
- Calories: 65

- Total Fat: 5g

- Carbohydrates: 4g

- Protein: 2g

- Fiber: 1g

- Sugar: 2g

Go ahead, treat yourself to one (or two!) of these pistachio delights. They're the perfect way to add a little green goodness and nutty flair to your Zepbound-friendly cookie lineup.

Chapter 21: Gingersnap Protein Cookies

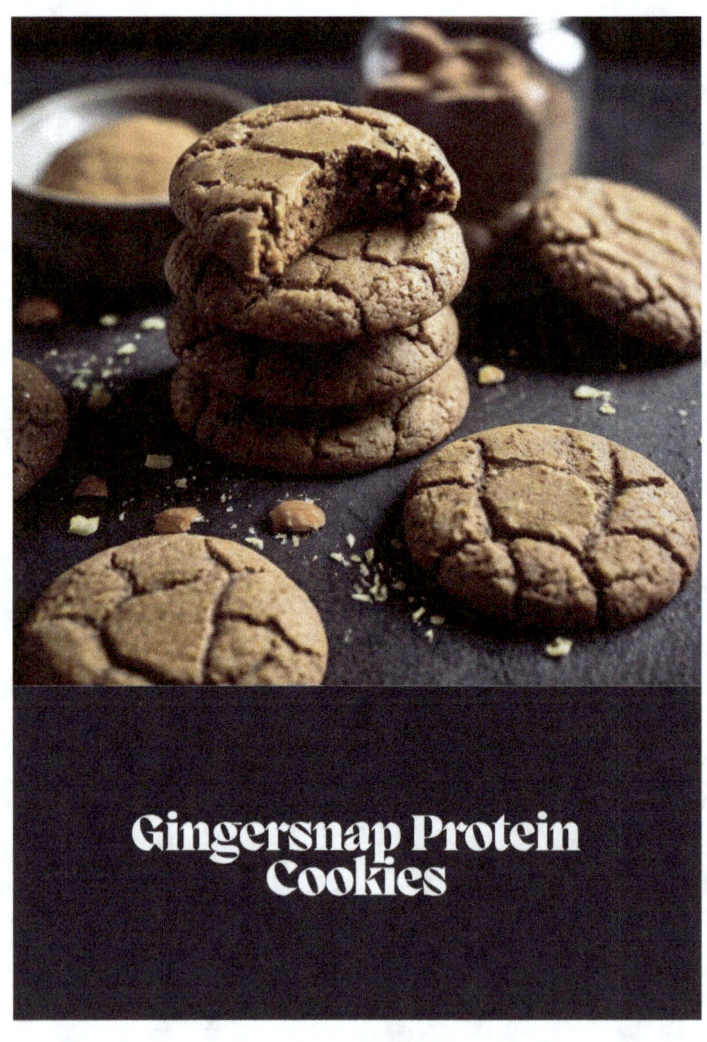

Now we're really talking about a cookie that's gonna keep you fueled and feeling fantastic! These little spicy-sweet bites are the perfect way to satisfy your sweet tooth while also giving your body a boost of protein.

Ingredients:

- 1/4 cup vanilla whey protein powder (the secret to packing in that extra punch of nutrition)
- 1 tbsp unsulfured molasses (just a touch, for that classic gingersnap flavor)
- 1 tsp ground ginger (because you can't have a gingersnap without the ginger!)
- 1 tbsp Monk fruit sweetener (to keep things Zepbound-friendly, of course)
- Pinch of salt (to really make those flavors pop)

Instructions:

1. Preheat your oven to a toasty 350°F (175°C) and line a baking sheet with parchment paper, because we all know how those pesky cookies can get a bit clingy if we don't give them a helping hand.

2. In a mixing bowl fit for a baking champion, combine the vanilla whey protein powder, unsulfured molasses, ground ginger, Monk fruit sweetener, and a pinch of salt. Mix it all together until it forms a delightfully spicy and protein-packed dough. It's like a little taste of the holidays, but with an added nutritional boost!

3. Scoop out the dough by the heaping tablespoonful and roll them into cute little rounds, about 1-inch in diameter. Arrange these precious gems on your prepared baking sheet, making sure to leave a smidge of space between each one - we don't want any cookie casualties!

4. Pop that tray into the oven and let the magic happen. Bake for 10-12 minutes, or until the edges are just starting to turn a lovely golden brown and the centers are still delightfully soft and chewy. It's like a little protein-packed hug for your taste buds in every bite!

5. Once they've had their time in the oven, remove the tray and let the cookies cool completely on the sheet.

This allows the centers to firm up just a touch, but still maintain that irresistible, melt-in-your-mouth texture.

Serving Size: 1-2 cookies

Nutritional Information (per 1 cookie):

- Calories: 50

- Total Fat: 1g

- Carbohydrates: 6g

- Protein: 4g

- Fiber: 1g

- Sugar: 2g

Conclusion

Hey bakers, as we finish up our cookie journey together I hope you feel nourished - both by these delicious recipes and the lessons they've taught! I know you've discovered the joy of baking treats that not only please your palate but also support your wellness goals. These cookies remind us it's not just about satisfying cravings - it's finding harmony in both body and soul through nourishment, connection and comfort. So whether you're hosting friends, gifting to loved ones or cozying up solo, I hope you feel these pages have brought some festive magic to your season.

Remember, the true spirit of holidays lies not in perfectly curated platters but in coming together through laughter and making memories. So let these Zepbound-friendly bakes be backdrops for cherished moments you'll hold dear for years to come.

Bake with care, share with warmth. Wishing you all the most wonderful cookie-filled celebrations and a bright, healthy new year ahead!

Thanks for joining me - it's been a sweet journey. Until next time, friends!